Ugonma Emeruem

Associations of Vigorous Physical Activity with Depression

AF190956

Ugonma Emeruem

Associations of Vigorous Physical Activity with Depression

An Examination of NHANES Data 2007-2008

LAP LAMBERT Academic Publishing

Imprint

Any brand names and product names mentioned in this book are subject to trademark, brand or patent protection and are trademarks or registered trademarks of their respective holders. The use of brand names, product names, common names, trade names, product descriptions etc. even without a particular marking in this work is in no way to be construed to mean that such names may be regarded as unrestricted in respect of trademark and brand protection legislation and could thus be used by anyone.

Cover image: www.ingimage.com

Publisher:
LAP LAMBERT Academic Publishing
is a trademark of
Dodo Books Indian Ocean Ltd. and OmniScriptum S.R.L publishing group

120 High Road, East Finchley, London, N2 9ED, United Kingdom
Str. Armeneasca 28/1, office 1, Chisinau MD-2012, Republic of Moldova, Europe
Managing Directors: Ieva Konstantinova, Victoria Ursu
info@omniscriptum.com

Printed at: see last page
ISBN: 978-3-659-41968-3

GEORGIA STATE UNIVERSITY

Associations of Vigorous Physical Activity with Depression: An Examination of
NHANES Data 2007-2008

Ugonma U. Emeruem

5/7/2013

Associations of Vigorous Physical Activity with Depression: An Examination of
NHANES Data 2007-2008

By

UGONMA ULOAKU EMERUEM

B.S., GEORGIA STATE UNIVERSITY

A Thesis submitted to the Graduate Faculty

Of Georgia State University in Partial Fulfillment

of the

Requirements for the Degree

MASTER OF PUBLIC HEALTH

ATLANTA GEORGIA

1

APPROVAL PAGE

Associations of Vigorous Physical Activity with Depression: An Examination of NHANES Data 2007-2008

by

UGONMA U. EMERUEM

Approved:

_____

Committee Chair

_____

Committee Member

_____

Committee Member

_____

DEDICATION PAGE

The following thesis document is dedicated to my family and loved ones.

ACKNOWLEDGEMENTS

I offer appreciation to my father and mother for financially supporting my degree and also for their kindness and freely given wisdom which has guided in my academic pursuits. I appreciate my siblings for their support through life's challenges. I would also like to acknowledge the staff and faculty of Georgia State University: Mrs. Courtney Burton, Mr. Bruce Perry, Mrs. Lisa Casanova and many others. I also acknowledge Francis Annor. Special thanks to thesis committee: Dr. Ike S. Okosun and Dr. Monic Swahn; I appreciate their support.

AUTHOR'S STATEMENT

In presenting this thesis as a partial fulfillment of the requirements for an advanced degree from Georgia State University, I agree that the Library of the University shall make it available for inspection and circulation in accordance with its regulations governing materials of this type. I agree that permission to quote from, to copy from, or to publish this thesis may be granted by the author or, in his/her absence, by the professor under whose direction it was written, or in his/her absence, by the Associate Dean, College of Health and Human Sciences. Such quoting, copying, or publishing must be solely for scholarly purposes and will not involve potential financial gain. It is understood that any copying from or publication of this dissertation which involves potential financial gain will not be allowed without written permission of the author.

_____
Signature of Author

5

Notice to Borrowers Page

All theses deposited in the Georgia State University Library must be used in accordance with the stipulations prescribed by the author in the preceding statement.
The author of this thesis is:
Student's Name: __UGONMA EMERUEM_____
Street Address: __300 PEACHTREE ST. NE, APT#
18G_____
City, State, and Zip Code: _____ATLANTA, GA,
30308_____
The Chair of the committee for this thesis is:
Professor's Name: IKE S. OKOSUN____ _____
Department: _____PUBLIC HEALTH_____ _____
College: _____INSTITUTE OF PUBLIC
HEALTH_____
Georgia State University
P.O. Box 3995
Atlanta, Georgia 30302-3995

Users of this thesis who not regularly enrolled as students at Georgia State University are required To attest acceptance of the preceding stipulation by signing below. Libraries borrowing this thesis for the use of their patrons are required to see that each user records here the

NAME OF USER	ADDRESS	DATE	TYPE OF USE (EXAMINATION ONLY OR COPYING)

CURRICULUM VITAE

Ugonma U. Emeruem

300 Peachtree St. NE, Apt# 18G   (404) 397-5152
Atlanta, GA 30308   uemeruem@gmail.com

OBJECTIVE: Internship involving public health based activities

EDUCATION

Georgia State University, Atlanta GA   Graduated 2008
B.S. in Biology, minor in Chemistry
GPA 3.4
Georgia State University, Atlanta GA   Expected graduation 2012
Masters in Public Health, concentration in Prevention Sciences
GPA 3.88

WORK EXPERIENCE
Georgia State University, Atlanta GA   1/2012-6/12
Graduate Research Assistant
- Assisted in gathering the professor's journal articles for research related to metabolic syndrome and analyzed data related to metabolic syndrome in people of West-African descent.
- Helped in the preparation of a Georgia State University online certificate Public Health program

Georgia State University, Atlanta GA   1/2007 – 5/07
Research/ Lab Assistant
- Provided research support in the study of the effect of agouti related protein administered in the paraventricular nucleus of the hypothalamus on appetitive behavior
- Contributed in the input of research data

Georgia State University Child Development Center, Atlanta GA   8/05 – 10/06
Student Assistant
- Provided assistance to the lead teacher in the education of toddlers
- Taught motor skills to toddlers

Children's Healthcare of Atlanta, Atlanta GA   7/05 – 12/06
Volunteer: Staff Assistant
- Organized and conducted children in-patient extracurricular activities at Hughes Spalding, Grady Memorial Hospital

SKILLS: Microsoft Office, SPSS

ABSTRACT

Background: Major depressive disorder or depression is a mental illness which affects people of a range of different ages. In terms of years lost due to disability, it is a leader. Physical activity is currently being used as a therapeutic treatment of depression that decreases levels of depression in individuals suffering from it. Physical activity can also be used as a form of prevention against depression. This study examines the association between vigorous physical activity and depression.

Methods: This is a cross-sectional study that utilized the secondary data from the National Health and Nutritional Examination Survey (NHANES) 2007-2008. Statistical Package for the Social Sciences (SPSS) is the software used in analyzing the descriptive data for the study. SAS was used for the logistic regression models. Univariate logistic regression was used to determine the association between physical activity and depression. A Multivariate analysis using SPSS determined the association between physical activity and depression adjusting for age, race, education, substance use, alcohol use, BMI and gender.

Results: The sample size for the cross-sectional study is 5553. The prevalence of depression in the different levels of physical activity are as follows: no physical activity (15.8%), insufficient physical activity (15.1%), moderate physical activity (12.8%), and vigorous physical activity (17.4%). The unadjusted odds ratio for the association between vigorous physical activity and depression is 1.15, and the adjusted odds ratio is 1.14. There is no significant association between vigorous physical activity and depression.

Conclusion: This study shows that there is no significant association between physical activity levels and depression. More research should be done to better understand the association between physical activity and depression.

TABLE OF CONTENTS

CHAPTER I

INTRODUCTION

1a. Current State of Depression

The International Classification of Disease (ICD) classify depressive disorders into four categories: - not depressed, mild depression; moderate depression and severe depression. Each degree of depression has a set number of symptoms amongst ten decisive key symptoms. The ten key symptoms are: persistent sadness; loss of interest; and fatigue for most days for a time of two weeks; Next, disturbed sleep; poor concentration or indecisiveness; low self-confidence, poor or increased appetite; suicidal thoughts or acts; agitation or slowing of movements, and guilt or self-blame (ICD-10 depression diagnostic criteria, 2013). The symptoms are summed up and the resultant number is tied to a classified degree.

In 2000, depression was the 4th leading contributor of the global burden of disease measured by Disability Adjusted Life Years (DALYs). Depression is projected to become 2nd overall in ranking for DALYs of all ages and both sexes and the 2nd leading cause of DALYs in the age category 15-44 years (Mental Health and Mental Health Disorders, 2011). Depression affects people of all ages; however, most studies show that people between the age of 45 and 64 experience major depression most frequently (Mental Health and Mental Health Disorders, 2011). Depression is the leading cause of disability measured in terms of Years Lost due to Disability (YLD) (Mental Health and Mental Health Disorders, 2011). Depression affects 121 million people in the world (Mental Health and Mental Health Disorders, 2011).

According to the CDC, 18.8 million American adults suffer from a depressive illness per year. Aforementioned, the problem of depression is considered the most prevalent mental health

10

problem in the older generation defined as individuals from the age 45 years and upward (Workplace Health Promotion, 2011). Depression is an insidious problem in the workplace, costing employers in the United States $17 billion to $44 billion (Workplace Health Promotion, 2011). The insidious nature of depression causes limitations in an employee's daily functioning which leads to an average of 4.8 missed work days, and 11.5 days of reduced productivity in a period of three months (Workplace Health Promotion, 2011). To combat the problem, Employers may offer costly mental health services such as visits to a therapist and medication (Workplace Health Promotion, 2011).

1b. Purpose of the Study

Physical activity improves the productivity of an individual suffering from depression (Lagerveld S.E. et al, 2010). A reduction in productivity is typically seen in employees in the workplace that suffer from depression (Workplace Health Promotion, 2011). Research by Lagerveld S.E. et al (2010) shows higher productivity levels from individuals suffering from depression when engaged in vigorous physical activity. This increase in productivity helps individuals suffering from depression in the work place by preventing job loss due to low work output (Lagerveld S.E. et al, 2010).

The current study is about the association between vigorous physical activity and depression. Healthy People 2020 have a topic area titled Mental Health and Mental Disorders. This topic area includes illnesses such as depression and anxiety. Mental Health is defined as a state of successful performance of mental function, resulting in productive activities, fulfilling relationships with other people, and ability to adapt to change and to cope with day by day challenge (Mental Health and Mental Health Disorders, 2011). This study examines the

11

relationship of physical activity with depression; a condition inhibits a person's ability to have fulfilling relationships with other people, ability to adapt to change and cope with day-to-day challenges (Mental Health and Mental Health Disorders, 2011). Understanding the association of physical activity on depression will help to determine if physical activity is a suitable intervention that can help improve the well-being of individuals suffering from depression.

Healthy People 2020 sees a connection between people's mental health and physical health (Mental Health and Mental Health Disorders, 2011). This connection is explored in this study by looking at the differences in the associations of different levels of physical activity and depression. How depression is affected by differing levels of physical activity can add to the understanding of the connection between a person's mental health and physical health by determining how higher or lower intensity physical activity levels affect a person's mental health; in this case, depression.

Physical activity is considered the health-promoting behavior in this study. The differences in the prevalence of physical activity engaged in depressed individuals and those who are not depressed can be explained by the Healthy People statement above.

Chronic disease can be a resulting outlook for an individual's ability to not participate in health-promoting behaviors (Mental Health and Mental Health Disorders, 2011). A lack of engagement in regular levels of physical activity by depressed individuals may indicate a possible neglect of other health promoting behaviors.

This study contributes to current and past research documents that study the association between physical activity and depression. It contributes to the literature by presenting the prevalence of physical activity among depressed persons; the prevalence information can then be used in proposing positive interventions in this demographic if it is needed. In addition, this study physical activity categorized into different levels. The finding will determine what category of physical activity has a stronger protective association with depression. The findings will be useful in designing physical activity interventions or prescriptions for depressed persons.

1c. Research Question

Question# 1: Is there an association between vigorous physical activity and depression in subjects in NHANES 2007-2008?

Null Hypothesis # 1: There is no association between vigorous physical activity and depression in subjects in NHANES 2007-2008.

Alternate Hypothesis # 1: There is an association between vigorous physical activity and depression in subjects in NHANES 2007-2008.

CHAPTER II

LITERRATURE REVIEW

The literature review is focused on understanding the disparities in the prevalence of depression among racial-ethnic groups as well as understanding the effect of physical activity on depression. Studies that discuss the level of productivity among individuals with depression are also noted. Finally the effect of different gradients of exercise on individuals suffering from depression is discussed.

2a. Physical Activity and Depression

Physical activity can be defined as movements performed by an individual that require more energy than when they are at rest (NHLBI, NIH, 2013). Exercise is a subset of physical activity that is planned, structured and repetitive for the purpose of conditioning the body (The Free Dictionary, n.d.).There is evidence that regular physical activity can lower your risk for early death, coronary heart disease, stroke, high blood pressure, high cholesterol or triglycerides, type 2 diabetes, metabolic syndrome, colon cancer, and breast cancer. It can also reduce the magnitude of symptoms experienced while depressed (CDC, 2008).

The intensity of physical activity can fluctuate from the insufficient physical activity which includes basic activities of daily living, and moderate to vigorous intensity. A moderate intensity physical activity is defined as an activity undergone by individual whereby the individual is unable to sing but can talk during the activity e.g. brisk walking, water aerobics, gardening. Vigorous intensity physical activity is defined as an activity undergone by individual in whom the person can barely speak e.g. jogging and jumping rope (CDC, 2008). Physical activity has been researched in relation to depression extensively when it comes to its therapeutic effects and some meta-analyses have shown that it seems to be an effective intervention for depression (Schuch et al, 2011). Some studies have proposed that the therapeutic effect of physical activity on individuals suffering from depression comes from the increased endorphin levels, increased self-esteem, and increased social interaction (Mikkelsen et al, 2010; Rot et al, 2009). Physical activity is also noted to affect an individual's central monoamine functioning (Mikkelsen et al, 2010). Single sessions of exercise can be beneficial in reducing depression symptoms but more sessions are even better (Rot et al, 2009) Several studies have shown an association between physical activity and a reduced risk of depressive symptoms (Lee.Y & Park K., 2008; Mikkelsen et al, 2010, Rot et al, 2009). Some studies show a link between recreational physical activity and reduced depression symptoms (Mikkelsen et al, 2010). Recreational physical activity is important in reducing depression symptoms in women. This relationship has a dose-response in men (Mikkelsen et al, 2010).

Physical activity is also important because older adults sometimes show a decline in physical function due to lifestyle changes and further knowledge about the added benefits of physical activity may be of additional importance. Information for improving disability related depressive symptoms is needed (Lee Y. & Park K., 2008). Physical activity can increase the Quality of Life (QOL) of individuals and even though its importance is stressed, whether or not physical activity is indeed a complementary strategy for the treatment of severe depression is still in question (Schuch F.B., 2011).

The researchers Beck, et al (2011) conducted a study that focused on depression, taking into account severity and loss of productivity for patients initiating treatment for their depression. The study used a heterogeneous population where patients were obtained from Depression Improvement Across Minnesota: Offering a New Direction (DIAMOND). Eight eight clinics and

23 medical groups participated in the study. The inclusion criteria involved patients that were older than 18 years and scored a 7 or higher on the Patient Health Questionnaire; a9-itemscreen (PHQ-9). Patients underwent baseline measures. The participants were followed for several months. A self-report questionnaire was used 6 months later which included PHQ-9 and a Work Productivity and Activity Impairment Questionnaire (WPAI). Covariates such as race, education, marital status and employment status were tested alongside PHQ-9 and were not found to be significant so were removed from the model. Minor levels of depression symptoms were associated with decreases in a person's work functioning (Beck A. et al, 2011).

There are studies done that examine the relationship between physical activity and depressive symptoms. A study conducted by Yunhwan Lee and Kyunghye Par which included data from Suwon Longitudinal Aging Study examined whether physical activity moderates the association between depressive symptoms and disability in community-dwelling older adults.. The subjects were randomly selected from a population registry. A Physical Functioning Scale, a Depression Scale and a Physical Performance test were used as measures in the study. Sociodemographic information was collected during the assessment. Cognitive function was assessed with a Mini-Mental State Examination. Cigarette smoking, alcohol drinking and body mass index were part of the data collected. The results showed that physical activity is an effect modifier of relationship between the depression symptoms and disability. Association between sociodemographic characteristics and health-related covariates were controlled for. Both moderate and vigorous physical activities were effective at reducing depressive symptoms. The authors noted that as time went on, the strength of association of this effect diminished (Lee Y. & Park K., 2008).

17

Another study investigated physical activity as an add-on for the treatment of severe depression with the intent of improving depressive symptoms and Quality of Life (QOL). The study was a randomized controlled trial with the control group receiving conventional treatments while the exercise group (or intervention group) received a physical exercise regimen that burnt 16kcals/kg/week during each of three sessions in addition to a conventional treatment regimen. After two weeks, results showed that both the exercise and control groups had marked improvement but the exercise group had an edge above the control group. QOL was also assessed to be higher in the exercise group than the control group, and therefore a decrease in depressive symptoms. One conclusion drawn was that exercise as an add-on for treatment is feasible and effective (Schuch et al, 2011).

Gamble, Ormerod, & Frenneaux, (2008) found exercise to be more beneficial at a higher intensity than a lower intensity, and saw that frequency of exercise was inconsequential. The inconsequentiality of longer exercise programs was also seen by authors Rethorst et al (2009). They saw that shorter interventions (4-9 weeks) were more beneficial that longer interventions (17-26 weeks). Rethorst et al (2009) study also saw results that verified the benefits of exercise, especially when they are a combination of aerobics and strength training. A 2009 Cochrane review also showed that a combination of aerobics and strength training termed 'mixed exercise' is more beneficial than aerobic exercise alone (Gill, Womack, & Safranek, 2010)

2b. Race and Depression

In the United States health care system, racial disparities are seen in the quality of care among individuals suffering from depression (Lukachko and Olfson, 2012). This disparity is typically seen in the primary care setting. The disparity is caused by underdiagnosing of depression in the African American patients when compared to Caucasians. This raises a problem for African Americans who tend to mostly utilize the primary care physicians for their mental health needs (Lukachko and Olfson, 2012). In addition, Skarupski et al (2005) states that African Americans when diagnosed have depressive symptoms that are more debilitating than other races. This is part of the reason why addressing the racial disparity issue concerning depression is a priority for public health professionals who aim to better the quality of care provided to individuals suffering from depression (Lukachko & Olfson, 2012).

A study conducted by Lukachko and Olfson (2012) depicted racial differences of depression diagnosis in office based primary care visits. Luckachko and Olson (2012) found that the African Americans were less likely to be diagnosed with depression during the primary care visits compared to Caucasians. Some of the factors driving this trend include cultural dissonance, mistrust and stigma that come with being seen as mentally ill in the medical setting. Stigma in the African American community will be addressed in more detail later in this document. Minorities and African Americans may bear the burden of these factors more than their Caucasian counterparts (Lukachko and Olfson, 2012). This racial disparity between African Americans and Caucasians causes problems for the African American community; Example of some of the problems include: late access to proper medication for African Americans due to underdiagnosed depression, and less productive individuals due to untreated depression

(Lukachko and Olfson, 2012). Lukachko and Olfson (2012) have suggested lessons on cultural

harmony for the primary care providers to HELPreduce this problem.

Table 1 illustrates the descriptive characteristics by race for the current level of

depression among adults in the United States, 2006 and 2008 (MMWR, 2010)

Table 1. An excerpt from the Weighted* percentage of adults meeting criteria for current depression,by type of depression and race — Behavioral Risk Factor Surveillance System, United States, 2006 and 2008

Race/Ethnicity	No in Sample	% Major Depression	95% CI Major Depression	% Other Depression	95% CI Other Depression	% Any current Depression	95% CI Any current Depression
Caucasian, non-Hispanic	183,563	3.1	2.9-3.2	4.8	4.6-5.0	7.9	7.6-8.1
African American, non-Hispanic	17,604	4.0	3.6-4.6	8.7	7.9-9.7	12.8	11.8-13.8
Hispanic	18,391	4.0	3.4-4.6	7.5	6.7-8.3	11.4	10.5-12.5
Other	13,528	4.3	3.6-5.1	6.3	5.5-7.3	10.6	9.5-11.9

Data were weighted to adjust for differences in probability of selection and nonresponse, as well as noncoverage (e.g., households lacking landlines).

As shown, Other races have the highest percentage of Major depression among all the

race. The next race to show high rates of depression is African American, non-Hispanic, and

Hispanic. The table shows disparity between the different races for depression.

Latzam et al (2011) states that previous studies on racial disparities in depression are

inconsistent. These authors explain that studies should be age group specific because the

prevalence of depression varies at different stages (Latzam et al, 2011). Latzam et al (2011) have conducted a cohort study on a diverse body of school children in the Southern United States to discern the racial differences in symptoms of depression among them. The Latzam et al (2011) study was unable to find statistically significant results for racial differences in symptoms of depression. (Latzam et al, 2011). A cross sectional study conducted by Weisbord et al (2007) also shows racial-ethnic differences in depression symptoms between Caucasian and African American. The severity of the symptoms is similar between Caucasian and African American. However, African Americans more than Caucasian use religion to cope with their illness (Weisbord, 2007).

With regards to Stigma, disparities between Caucasians and ethnic minorities such as African Americans and Hispanics can be attributed to stigma which affects the ethnic minorities (Fleming et al, 2011). A cross sectional study by Fleming et al (2001) showed that out of their participants, Caucasians suffering from major depression where most likely to have been taking medication. The chi-square analysis frequency rate was 37.6%, followed by Hispanic with a usage rate of 21.8%, and finally African Americans with 17.5%. However, when the results were adjusted with covariates such as gender, age, income, education, marital status, and work status they were no longer significant. The range for acceptance of antidepressants among Minorities in the United States is one-third to one-half. African Americans and Hispanics have self-hindering beliefs that deter them from taking antidepressants. Examples include the belief that anti-depressants are addictive and religious activities such as prayer are most likely the cure (Fleming et al, 2011). Stigma is seen among Caucasians when friends and family become involved in the treatment process (Fleming et al, 2011).Stigma concerning depression in the ethnic minority communities contributes to the lower rates of taking medication (Fleming et al, 2011).

Treatment for depression includes: Selective serotonin reuptake inhibitors (SSRIs), serotonin norepinephrine reuptake inhibitors (SNRIS), Mirtazapine or Bupripone (Fleming, Barner, Brown & Smith, 2011). However, having readily available drugs are rendered useless if the individuals meant to take them do not take the medications or have access to it. Some causes of lack of access and usage are underdiagnoses in minority communities, (Fleming et al, 2011; Lukachko and Olfson, 2012), misdiagnosis, stigma and patients beliefs (Fleming et al, 2011). African Americans and Hispanic are most affected by these causes and are 50% less likely than Causcasians to get treated for their depression.

African American adults who are over 65 years are less likely to seek out treatment for their depression than their Caucasian counter parts. Moreover, African American older adults who are on a treatment regimen often have been found not to complete their treatment (Conner et al, 2010). Some unique barriers faced by African American older adults and Hispanic older adults include ageism (belief that you are too old to be treated), fear and distrust of the health care system, lack of information, no insurance, and no transport to health care institutions (Conner et al, 2010). Negative beliefs toward mental health in general are also a problem (Conner et al, 2010; Fleming et al, 2011). Conner et al (2010) conducted 37 interviews of older African American adults and discovered some beliefs that hinder treatment of depression in the African American community. Some of the belief include: lack of tolerance for mental health issues, secrecy, fear of being stigmatized for life because you had the illness, and fear of being "African American and depressed", internalized stigma, and ignorance within the community. Beliefs create a lot of barriers for African Americans to receive the help they need (Conner et al, 2010).

Depression rates among Latino immigrants tend to increase the longer they reside in the United States. Some of the increase can be attributed to pre-migration, migration and post-migration experiences. Entering the United States, major life events and coming from poverty contributed to pre-migration stress, racial discrimination is the major stressor thereafter (Ornelas, & Perreira, 2011).

Asians reportedly have the lowest lifetime prevalence of major depression, and this prevalence is even lower in Asians not born in the United States, but still greater than Asians residing abroad. (Kalibatseva & Leong, 2011). When Asian Americans get depressed, they are less likely to seek treatment or be diagnosed compared to non-Hispanic Caucasians (Kalibatseva & Leong, 2011).

2c. Age and Depression

Nguyen and Zonderman (2006) acknowledge the discrepancy between various studies on the connection between age and depression. Researchers on this subject have come to very different conclusions. Researchers have presented conflicting results regarding which age group has the highest prevalence of depression. Some studies say that young adults have the highest frequency of depression. Others say that depression is most prevalent in the elderly population. In regards to the middle-aged population, researchers have also presented varied results: some find that depression increases during middle age, other studies show that depression neutralizes in this same age group. A sample of National Center for Health Statistics (NHANES) for psychological data 1971 to 1975 is used by Nguyen and Zonderman (2006) to research whether depression has a relationship to age. Center for Epidemiological Studies Depression Scale (CES-

D) was the instrument used to measure depression in this cross-sectional study. The results

showed that depressed mood was not affected by age (Nguyen and Zonderman, 2006).

About 20 percent of the adolescent population in the United States suffers from

Depression (Cook, Peterson, & Sheldon, 2009). Two percent of children ages 6 to 12 suffer from

major depression (Cook, Peterson, & Sheldon, 2009). Sometimes the disease is undetected in

adolescence because it is mistaken for teenage angst or moodiness. It causes some functional

impairment and hinders normal psychosocial development (Cook, Peterson, & Sheldon, 2009).

The mean onset of major depression in adolescents is 14.9 years (Lewinsohn, Rohde, & Seeley,

1998). Timing of puberty is related to depression rates in adolescent girls while insignificant in

adolescent boys (Lewinsohn, Rohde, & Seeley, 1998). Some studies suggest screening for

depression in adolescents and gearing consequent therapy towards their needs (Cook, Peterson,

&Sheldon, 2009: Lewinsohn, Rohde, & Seeley, 1998). Indirect and open-ended questions are

critical when screening adolescents as they may not be able to articulate their feelings properly

(Cook et al, 2009). Dysphoric mood, poor self-esteem, interpersonal difficulties, and coping

techniques are common areas that teens who seek therapy are hoping to address (Lewinsohn,

Rohde, & Seeley, 1998).

Untreated depression in adolescents may lead to attempted suicide, which occurs in 30

percent of adolescents suffering from major depression (Cook et al, 2009). Some studies state

that substance abuse is also an issue with Adolescents suffering from depression (Audrain-

McGovern, Rodriguez, & Kassel, 2009; Cook et al 2009). Audrain-McGovern et al (2009) study

indicates that the nature of depression leaves the adolescent more susceptible to smoking.

Adolescent onset depression tends to be more severe than Adult onset depression (Cook,

24

Peterson & Sheldon, 2009). Adolescent depression can also persist into adulthood (Cook, Peterson & Sheldon, 2009).

Middle aged individuals suffering from depression have poorer health-related quality of life and are more likely to have work-related disability (Covinsky et al, 2010).Covinsky et al (2010) studies whether middle age individuals suffering from depression are more likely to suffer from disability in their elderly years This was a prospective study with a twelve year follow up. Over the twelve years there was a statistically significant result (Hazard Ratio =1.44, 95% CI=1.25-1.66) which showed that middle aged individuals suffering from depression are more likely to have some disability associated with Activities of Daily Living (ADL), and mobility difficulty in their elderly years. Interventions focused on preventing the middle age from developing disability in their elderly years by screening for depression during their middle aged years have not yet been proven to be effective. This is because of treatment of depression in middle age has not been shown to prevent disability in the elderly years (Covinsky et al, 2010).

Self-transcendence is an important part of middle age mental health. Self-transcendence is a process whereby an individual pushes the boundaries of their lives (Ellermann & Reed, 2001). The boundaries that are pushed in the lives of the middle age are physical and existential in nature. The boundaries manifest physically through relationships which are familial and peer related, success. Existentially it pertains to spirituality. During the middle age years women depression rates (2.9% to 5.2%) are double that of men's depression rates (.1.6% to 3.2%) (Ellermann & Reed, 2001). Ellermann and Reed (2001) showed in their study the more self-transcendent a middle aged adult was the less likely they were to suffer from depression. When the physical boundary of parenting is pushed, parenting in terms of number of children being raised, is pushed, there is an inverse relationship with depression. In addition, the higher the

25

levels of self-acceptance in the middle age years lead to lower the likelihood of depression. The results listed so far are statistically significant with r=.51, p<.001 for the relationship between self-transcendence and depression (Ellermann & Reed, 2001).

Table 2 illustrates the descriptive characteristics for current Depression among different age groups in the United States, 2006 and 2008 (MMWR, 2010).

Table2. Weighted* percentage of adults meeting criteria for current depression,† by type of depression and age — Behavioral Risk Factor Surveillance System, United States, 2006 and 2008

Age group	No. in sample	Major Depression %	Major Depression 95% CI	Other Depression %	Other Depression 95% CI	Any current depression %	Any current depression (95% CI)
18-24	9944	2.8	2.3-3.4	8.1	7.2-9.2	10.9	9.8-12.1
25-34	27,086	3.4	3.0-3.9	5.6	5.2-6.2	9.1	8.5-9.8
35-44	39,440	3.6	3.2-4.0	5.0	4.7-5.5	8.6	8.1-9.2
45-64	97,642	4.6	4.3-5.0	5.4	5.0-5.8	10.0	9.5-10.5
>=65	59,246	1.6	1.4-1.8	5.2	4.9-5.6	6.8	6.4-7.2

*Data were weighted to adjust for differences in probability of selection and nonresponse, as well as noncoverage (e.g., households lacking landlines).

The subpopulation of interest is Age group 45-64 and those suffering from Major Depression. Out of 97,642 people in this age group, 4.9% (CI: 4.3-5.0) suffer from major depression. 4.7(CI: 5.0-5.8) suffer from other depression, and 9.6 (CI: 9.5-10.5) suffer from any depression (MMWR, 2010). This age group is describe in most studies as having the highest prevalence of depression out of the different age groups.

Older Americans (age 65 years and older) make up 12% of the United States population, 16%of suicides in the United States come from this population. 14.3 per 100,000 older adults committed suicide in 2001. Non-Hispanic Caucasian men age 85 yearsand older have a high

suicide rate of 49.8 per 100,000. Asian and Pacific Islanders have a rate of 10.6 per 100,000,

Hispanics have a rate of 7.9 per 100,000 and Non-Hispanic African Americans have a rate of 5.0

per 100,000. Depression is mistaken in this population as a normal part of ageing. Depression

also tends to occur with other medical illnesses in these populations and can cause a slower

recovery in both illnesses (NIMH, 2003).

2d. Gender and Depression

A consistent finding in studies is that depression is more prevalent among women

compared to men (Essau et al, 2010; Miller et al, 2011; Velde, Bracke, & Levecque, 2010;

Velde, Bracke, Levecque, & Bart, 2010). This gender difference is seen in adolescent years and

adulthood (Essau et al, 2010). The gender difference begins at age 11 for girls, which marks the

onset of puberty (Miller et al, 2011). The biggest gender gap occurs between the ages 15 and 18,

and the possible reasons include changes in hormones, stress and differences in socialization

(Essau et al, 2010). This gender difference is also seen in the area of recurrence of a depressive

episode for those with a past history of depression. However, the opinion on recurrence is

unclear because some cases show women suffer higher recurrences than men, other say men

suffer more and some say there is no difference (Essau et al, 2010; Miller et al, 2011).

The table below describes on a National level, the percentages by classification of

depression by gender for Depression in the United States. There are 89,842 male with a

prevalence of 3.3 (CI: 3.0-3.5) suffering from major depression, and 145, 225 female with a prevalence of 4.8 (CI: 4.6-5.1) showing that more women suffer from depression than men

(MMWR, 2010).

Table 3. Weighted* percentage of adults meeting criteria for current depression by type of

depression and gender— Behavioral Risk Factor Surveillance System, United States, 2006 and

2008

Gender	No. in Sample	Major Depression %	Major Depression (95% CI)	Other Depression %	Other Depression (95% CI)	Any current depression %	Any current depression (95% CI)
Men	89,842	2.7	2.5-3.0	5.2	4.9-5.5	7.9	7.5-8.2
Women	145,225	4.0	3.8-4.2	6.1	5.9-6.4	10.1	9.8-10.4

* Data were weighted to adjust for differences in probability of selection and nonresponse, as well as noncoverage (e.g., households lacking landlines).

Some explanations for this phenomenon of women being more depressed is the role and

limitations that society sometimes places on them. Modern married women have to be supportive

wives, primary caretakers of the children, and bring income. Stay-at-home moms are becoming

undervalued. They face discrimination at work, and this hurts them economically (Velde, Bracke

& Levecque, 2010). Velde et al (2010) found in their study that marriage is a buffer against

depression for both men and women.

Menstrual cycles bring about hormonal changes in women which can cause mood

changes. Post-partum depression occurs after some women have given birth. Women also face

more violence e.g. sexual abuse and domestic abuse. Some of the abuse can happen in the early

stages of their lives and have devastating effects on their mental health (Miller et al, 2011

2e. Depression and Productivity

Several studies have mentioned depression as very costly to jobs with respect to the employer but also for the employee with depression (Eldin, 2006; Durr, 2011; Lagerveld S.E. et al, 2010; Marlowe, 2002). The stress on current work environments has led to the increase in the amount of depressed employees. However, mental health expenditures have decreased because hospitals have shifted of the mental health care to out-patient services (Marlowe, 2002). Cost of loss of productivity due to mental illness can be in measured by using lost wages and/ or substandard work produced for the employer (Lagerveld S.E. et al, 2010). Substandard work is caused by worker impairment, and the behavior is called Presenteeism. Presenteeism can be worse than a worker being absent (Marlowe, 2002). Even when depressed patients are receiving correct treatment some health care practitioners may not permit them to go to work because they believe the job is part of their patients' problem (Marlowe, 2002).

Individuals suffering from depression are usually unaware that they need help and can get help. This lets the insidious problem of presenteeism to pervade. Individuals suffering from depression are 23% less productive than they can be. These individuals tend to feel hopeless and take more sick leaves (Edlin, 2006). Depression can also be a comorbid condition (Edlin, 2006; Marlowe, 2002). Twenty five percent of cancer patients can expect depression as a comorbid condition along with their illness, twenty five percent of myocardial infraction patents will have depression as a comorbidity, depression is experienced by seventy five percent of chronic fatigue syndrome patients (Marlowe, 2002).

Work disability has been shown to have a strong relationship with a long duration of a depressive episode; this in terms of work participation may indicate work status and days at work

(Lagerveld S.E. et al, 2010). There is some evidence that shows an association between severe depressive disorder and work disability, however, this association was shown in older adults, history of previous sick leave and presence of mental and physical comorbidities (Lagerveld S.E. et al, 2010). For work functioning, severe depressive symptoms were related to work productivity (Lagerveld S.E. et al, 2010). According to Beck et al (2011), several studies have demonstrated an association between depression and work disability or performance. Some have shown a continuum of severity of the depression to the amount of work lost. E.g. an increase in symptoms severity is associated with numbers of days absent at work due to depression. Some of the factors that translate depression as a work disability are productivity, decrease in work quality, mistakes and errors, work accidents, more sick leaves, disability pensions and unfavorable career perspectives. Lagerveld S.E. et al (2010) sum all these factors under the terms "Work Participation" and "Work Functioning".

Lagerveld S.E. et al (2010) define work participation as the capability and/or opportunity to participate in the workforce, fulfilling one's work role. Lack in work participation can lead to absenteeism, early retirement and employment termination. Comparisons done clinically have shown that depressed individuals have a longer duration of absence due to sickness than non-depressed individuals. Work functioning is defined by Lagerveld S.E. et al (2010) as the productivity or performance of employees that participate, at least partly, in work, and is the result of a relationship between an individual's health resources and the expectations and structural conditions that operate within social settings such as the work place. Depression has been associated with a decrease in work functioning through work productivity and increasing work limitations. Individuals with depression have to put forth extra effort to deliver work that is acceptable (Lagerveld S.E. et al, 2010).

30

The evidence that links depression to a depreciated work performance leads to questions about possible interventions. Worker-directed 'clinical' interventions effectiveness was reviewed through a search of the Cochrane Reviews; however the search produced limited results. The search produced limited amount of results on this issue and this in itself is evidence that there is a strong need to evaluate and develop interventions that will increase work functioning and work participation in depressed workers (Lagerveld S.E. et al, 2010). Knowledge of the factors that influence work participation and work functioning are important in developing interventions related to this issue. However, this knowledge is still relatively unclear, but some people have attempted to clarify this issue. A multidisciplinary expert group, using the WHO ICF model, discovered some possible predictive modifiable factors e.g. coping/appraisal, self-efficacy, professional competence and perfectionism (Lagerveld S.E. et al, 2010). Modifiable risk factors are those risk factors that can be realistically changed through intervention. Some work environment factors that may be modifiable include work demands, workplace culture, social support, and job security and decision latitude.

CHAPTER III

METHODOLOGY

3a. Data Source

The secondary data used in this study is from the National Health and Nutrition Examination Survey (NHANES). NHANES, is conducted by the National Center for Health Statistics (NCHS) which is part of the Center for Disease Control and Prevention (CDC) and it is responsible for providing vital and health statistics for the United States. Children and adults are assessed in this survey, and this assessment includes interviews and physical examination (CDC, 2012). The NHANES studies began in the early 1960s.Demographic, socioeconomic, dietary, laboratory tests, physiological measurements, medical, dental and health-related questions are collected. The 2007-2008 NHANES data was used in this cross-sectional study. To select a participant, NHANES used a statistical process to divide the United States into communities that are then further divided into neighborhoods. Each participant's identity is kept confidential. Each neighborhood has houses units from which eligible housing units are randomly selected (NHANES, 2013).

The National Health Survey Act, 1956 is the parent of NHANES. The law laid provisions for a survey to collect statistical data on the amount, distribution and effects of illness and disability in the United States. The NHANES survey is conducted by professional individuals from varied backgrounds such as social work, the military, education, medical doctors, nurses, health educators, engineers and doctoral degree holders. The reports of their tests are also mailed to the participants. Finally a cash payment for participating in the survey is given. Participants are expected to participate in an interview process that is done by an interviewer at home and also by an online interview, and a health examination in a Mobile Exam center (NHANES, 2013).

NHANES 2007-2010 sampling methodology involved the oversampling of Hispanics which include more than Mexican Americans. They also combined the age range of 12-15 to 16-19, and split the age range of 40-50 to 40-49 and 50-59. Pregnant women were not oversampled. These changes led to some variable being modified. In earlier years low income persons, adolescents, the elderly, African Americans, and Mexican American were over-sampled. In the year 2012 some additional tests were included (NHANES, 2013). Some of the questions asked in the NHANES 2007-2008 survey have been asked in previous NHANES surveys dating from 1976-1980, 1982-84, 1988-1994 and 1999- 2006 (NHANES, 2013).

NHANES 2006-2007 data set depression screener questions are based on a Prime-MD diagnostic instrument (NHANES, 2013). Physical activity is measured with a Global Physical Activity Questionnaire (GPAQ).

3b. Inclusion and Exclusion Criteria

The sample (n=5553) for this study consisted of people from the NHANES 2007-2008 data that were aged 20 years or more.

Demographic Variables

The demographic variables included in the study were RIAGENDR (gender), (RIAAGEYR) age and RIDRETH1 (race/ethnicity). Other demographic variables and sample weight files were removed. Eligible subjects for this analysis had values on age, ethnicity and gender questions and those with missing values were excluded.

Age is a continuous variable and is categorized and coded into groups as follows: Age: 20-29=1, 30-39= 2, 40-49= 3, 50-59=4, 60-69= 5. Gender variables for male is coded as 1 while Gender variable for female is coded as 2. The ethnicity variables were coded into '1' equals Non-Hispanic White, '2' equals Other Hispanic, '3' equals Mexican American, '4' equals Non-Hispanic Black and '5' Other.

Dependent Variable

Depression is the independent Variable in this study. The questionnaire tilted "Depression Screener" from NHANES 2007-2008 was used to define depression in this study. People that did not answer questions from the depression screener in its entirety were excluded from the study. Respondents that gave a positive response for at least five of the questions below were categorized as having Major Depression.

I. Little interest in doing things?

II. Feeling down, depressed, or hopeless?

III. Trouble sleeping or sleeping too much?

IV. Feeling tired or having little energy?

V. Poor appetite or overeating?

VI. Feeling bad about yourself?

VII. Trouble concentrating on things?

VIII. Moving or speaking slowly or too fast?

IX. Thought you would be better off dead?

Independent Variables

Physical activity measure was obtained from the Physical Activity questionnaire file from NHANES 2007-2008. Physical activity was categorized into no physical activity, insufficient physical activity, moderate physical activity and vigorous physical activity. Vigorous physical activity was derived from the question "days vigorous recreational activities"; those with greater than three days a week of vigorous recreational activities where labeled vigorously active. Moderate physical activity was derived from the question "days moderate recreational activities"; those with greater than five days were defined as having moderate physical activity. Insufficient physical activity was defined that did engage in physical activity but that at the recommended levels. No physical activity is defined as people that did not engage in physical activity. The definitions for vigorous physical active, insufficient physical activity, and moderate physical activity were gotten from CDC (CDC, 2013).

Body Mass Index (BMI) was calculated with the study population weight in pounds and height in inches. The categories for BMI are underweight, normal, overweight and obese. Substance use was derived from the question: Ever used cocaine/heroin/methamphetamine? Substance use was categorized into users and non-users. Alcohol use was categorized into normal, heavy, and binge. The CDC defines normal alcohol use as one drink a day for women and two drinks a day for men. Heavy drinkers are defined as females that drink more than one drink a day and males that drink more than two drinks a day. Binge drinkers are defined as four or more drinks a day for women and five or more drinks a day for men (CDC 2013). Education was categorized as less than high school, high school graduate, some college and college graduate. The questions in NHANES specified the education level categories.

3c. Statistical Procedure

Statistical Package for the Social Sciences (SPSS) was used in setting up the data. Descriptive statistics was derived for the demographic variables using SPSS. Prevalence of depression among the different independent variables was obtained. SAS was used to run univariate logistic regression to determine the association between physical activity level and depression. Multivariate analysis association between physical activity level and depression was done adjusting for age, race, gender, education, substance use, BMI and alcohol use.

CHAPTER IV

RESULTS

4a. Descriptive Statistics

The sample size for the study population is 5553. The demographics characteristics of the respondents in this study with respect to gender, race/ethnicity and age are included in Table 4. Majority of the respondents were between the ages 30-39 (25.1%). Non-Hispanic white represented 40.5% of the respondents.

Table 4: Demographic Characteristics of Study Population (n=5553)

Variable	Percent	95% CI
Gender		
Male	49.8	48.5-51.1
Female	50.2	48.9-51.5
Race/Ethnicity		
Non-Hispanic White	40.5	39.2-41.8
Non-Hispanic Black	21.8	20.7-22.8
Mexican American	21.6	20.5-22.7
Other Hispanic	11.5	10.7-12.3
Other	4.6	4.1-5.2
Age (Years)		
20-29	16.4	15.4-17.3
30-39	25.1	24.0-26.2
40-49	21.2	20.1-22.3
50-59	14.1	13.2-15.1
60-69	11.1	10.2-11.9
70+	12.1	11.3-13.0

Table 5 represents the distribution of the dependent variable depression, and the

independent variables such as substance use, BMI, alcohol use, physical activity. 66.1% of the

study respondents represent the no physical activity category. 84.5% of the study population is

not depressed. Normal alcohol users represent 69.5% of the study population. Respondent with

less than high school education represent 30.9% of the study population.

Table 5: Distribution of Dependent and Independent Factors

Variable	Percent	95% CI
Substance Use		
Non-User	87.7	86.8-88.5
User	12.3	11.5-13.2
BMI		
Under Weight	3.8	3.3-4.3
Normal Weight	32.0	30.8-33.2
Over Weight	34.0	32.7-35.3
Obese	30.2	28.9-31.4
Alcohol Use		
Normal	69.5	68.3-70.7
Heavy	21.6	20.5-22.7
Binge	8.9	8.1-9.6
Depression		
Depressed	84.5	83.6-85.5
Not Depressed	15.5	14.5-16.4
Physical Activity		
No Physical Activity	66.1	64.9-67.4
Insufficient	20.8	19.7-21.9
Moderate	8.0	7.3-8.7
Vigorous	5.1	4.5-5.6
Education		
Less than High School	30.9	29.7-32.15
High School Grad	25.0	23.9-26.19
Some College	25.9	24.7-27.04
College Graduate	18.1	17.1-19.1

4b. Prevalence

"Other races" experience the highest prevalence (18.2%) of depression. Females had a statistically significantly higher prevalence of depression than males. Age group 50-59 had the highest prevalence 17.7 of depression. These results are statistically significant according to the 95% CI.

Table 6: Prevalence of Depression by Demographic Characteristics

Demographic Characteristics	%Prevalence of Depression	95% CI
Gender		
Male	15.1	13.7-16.4
Female	15.9	14.5-17.2
Race/Ethnicity		
Non-Hispanic White	14.9	13.4-16.3
Non-Hispanic Black	15.1	13.0-17.1
Mexican American	15.2	13.1-17.2
Other Hispanic	17.9	14.9-20.8
Other	18.2	13.5-23.0
Age (Years)		
20-29	15.0	12.6-17.3
30-39	16.2	14.3-18.1
40-49	15.3	13.2-17.4
50-59	17.7	15.0-20.4
60-69	13.5	10.8-16.2
70+	14.1	11.5-16.8

The prevalence of depression in category non-users for substance use is 15.5%. Underweight respondents have the highest prevalence (20.5%) of depression in the BMI category. Depression Prevalence by physical activity showed that individuals who engaged in vigorous physical activity have a prevalence of 17.4%. Complete results of prevalence of depression by independent variables are shown in Table 7.

Table 7: Prevalence of Depression by the Independent variables

Variables	Prevalence of Depression	95% CI
Substance Use		
Non-User	15.5	14.5-16.5
User	15.1	12.4-17.7
BMI		
Under Weight	20.5	15.0-26.0
Normal Weight	15.8	14.1-17.5
Over Weight	14.6	13.0-16.2
Obese	15.6	13.9-17.4
Alcohol Use		
Normal	15.2	14.1-16.3
Heavy	16.6	14.5-18.7
Binge	14.8	11.6-17.9
Education		
Less than High School	15.1	13.4-16.8
High School Grad	15.0	13.1-16.9
Some College	16.6	14.7-18.5
College Graduate	15.0	12.8-17.2
Physical Activity		
No Physical Activity	15.8	14.6-16.9
Insufficient	15.1	13.0-17.1
Moderate	12.8	9.7-16.0
Vigorous	17.4	13.0-21.9

4c Depression and Physical Activity Level Association

The results of the univariate and multivariate analysis of the association between physical activity level and depression is shown in Table 8. Odds ratio from the logistic regression models are used to quantify the magnitude of association. There is no significant association between physical activity level and depression.

Table 8: Association between Physical Activity and Depression

Physical Activity Level	Crude Odds Ratio	95% CI	Adjusted Odds Ratio	95% CI
No Physical Activity	Ref	Ref	Ref	Ref
Insufficient	0.95	0.79-1.15	0.95	0.79-1.15
Moderate	0.78	0.58-1.05	0.79	0.59-1.06
Vigorous	1.15	0.83-1.59	1.14	0.82-1.57

Note: The adjusted Odds Ratio has adjusted for Sex, Age, Race, Education, Substance use, BMI, and Alcohol use

CHAPTER V

DISCUSSION AND CONCLUSION

The study objective was to research the association between vigorous physical activity and depression in subjects in NHANES 2007-2008. The odd ratio 1.14 from the multivariate analysis in this study shows a positive association between vigorous physical activity and depression. A negative association with depression is seen in individuals that engage in moderate physical activity. According to Song et al (2011) moderate physical activity group showed people with less likelihood to have depression. Insufficient physical activity also has a negative association with depression. However, the results in this study are not statistically significant.

Similar studies show that Individuals engaged in vigorous physical activity are less likely to be depressed (Harris, Cronkite & Moss, 2006). Harris, Cronkite and Moss (2006) adjusted for gender, age, and physical disability in their study and arrived at the conclusion that individuals engaged in moderate physical activity have higher odds of depression compared to individuals engaged in vigorous physical activity; this is inconsistent with this study which finds vigorous physical activity associated with increased likelihood of depression though insignificant.

In this study, 60-69 year olds had the lowest prevalence of depression. Normal aging brings with it a decrease in physical function but this physical function should not affect an individual's quality of life (Fukukawa et al, 2004).. According to Fukukawa et al (2004), family support buffers the decline of physical activity in the elderly and also buffers the incidence of depressive symptoms in the middle age. Questions about social support can be included in future studies concerning depression and physical activity in older adults. Individuals that had family members living with them might have had lower levels of depression.

42

In this study, women have a significantly higher prevalence (15.9%) of depression compared to men. Childless mothers reported having significantly higher levels of depression than mothers who were childless by choice, and those who have children. Stigma associated with childlessness plague some women more than others. The higher percentage of depression in women in this present study can be attributed to this problem (Koropeckyj-Cox, 1998). Post-menopausal women have increased risks of depression (Gibbs, Lee & Kulkarni, 2010). This study remains consistent with other studies that show that depression is more prevalent in women (Essau et al, 2010; Miller et al, 2011; Velde, Bracke, & Levecque, 2010; Velde, Bracke, Levecque, & Bart, 2010).

Substance non-users have a higher prevalence (15.5%) of depression than substance users in this study. The prevalence of depression in substance users is 15.1%. Substance use tends to be comorbid with depression (Swendsen & Merikangas, 2000). It would be expected that substance users would have a higher prevalence of depression when compared to substance non-users but this is not the case here. People use hard drugs have higher depressive symptoms (Illangasekare et al, 2013). There could have been underreporting of depressive symptoms by the Substance users in this study which could serve as a reason for this difference. In addition the proportion of Substance non-users is much higher than the proportion of substance users in this study. This unbalanced proportion could have made it possible for more depressed individuals to be included in the overall number of substance non users.

There is an increase in the prevalence of depression in those who drink alcohol normally (15.2%) to those who drink alcohol heavily (16.6%). Literature shows a causal relationship between depression and alcohol use. The relationship between alcohol and depression can be in terms of increased alcohol usage increases risk of depression or depression increases risk of alcohol use (Boden & Fergusson, 2010). Binge drinkers in this study have the lowest prevalence of depression. Alcohol may be used by this group to self-medicate the symptoms of depression and that result in underreported symptoms of depression (Boden & Fergusson, 2010). A future study can break down alcohol usage categories by gender to note possible differences (Boden & Fergusson, 2010).

"Other race" has the highest prevalence of depression. This finding is coincides with the data in the Mortality and Morbidity Weekly Report titled Current Depression Among Adults --- United States, 2006 and 2008 (MMWR, 2010). Other Hispanic had the second highest prevalence of depression. Mexican American and Non-Hispanic Black had higher depression prevalence levels when compared to Non-Hispanic White which had the lowest prevalence of depression. These results are similar to other studies (MMWR, 2010; Latino MH Facts, 2013)

The underweight BMI category has the highest prevalence (20.5%) of depression. The depression prevalence decreases in the normal category and decreases further in the overweight category before increasing in the Obese. Underweight people have the highest prevalence of depression (Wit et al, 2009). It is typical to see a decrease in depression prevalence when moving from the underweight category to the normal category (Wit et al, 2009). Higher education level protects against depression (Bjelland et al, 2008). In this study College graduate have a one of the lowest prevalence of depression (15.0%). However, the relationship between the prevalence of depression and education level is not linear in this study. Respondents in the category some college have the highest prevalence of depression (16.6%). Some of the respondents in this category could have been college dropouts and their inclusion in the category could have skewed the results.

Limitations

This is a cross-sectional study that uses secondary data. Cross-sectional studies do not show causation because they take only a snap shot at a point in time of the independent and outcome variable. In addition, secondary data has a problem of not being tailor-made to answer the questions proposed by the researcher utilizing them. The secondary data is from NHANES 2007-2008 and is self-reported. There could be self-reporting bias involved. In this present study there is no distinction between the individuals who are suffering from depression and taking medication for depression and those individuals who are suffering from depression and not taking depression medication. This study may be biased in terms of prevalence.

Recommendations

Physical activity interventions are being seen as an important intervention when it comes to depression and as a different option to drug therapy. Individuals who took their usual drug therapy medication for depression and engaged in a physical activity treatment of depression reported increased rates of physical activity overall (Chalder et al, 2012). More research should be done to understand the association between physical activity and depression.

Conclusion

This study is important because it provides the prevalence of depression among a national sample of individuals. The prevalence of depression varies across the different categories of the independent variables. These results are useful for the public health community in developing health promotion solutions to depression in the United States. For example, the prevalence of depression in the different race/ethnicity categories is consistent with past literature and these

45

results can strengthen grant queries for interventions concerning race and depression. In addition, the substance users have a lower prevalence of depression when compared to substance non-users can help public health professionals make surveys on depression that ask if the person is self-medicates negative feelings with drugs. That question can change the way the respondent would answers subsequent question about depressive symptoms because he or she would recall the state they are typically in before they have self-medicated and answer the questions accordingly. This study shows that there is no significant association between physical activity and depression.

REFERENCES

Aan het Rot, Marije, Katherine A Collins, and Heidi L Fitterling. "Physical Exercise and Depression."
The Mount Sinai Journal of Medicine, New York 76, no. 2 (April 2009): 204–214.

Beck, A, AL Crain, LI Solberg, J Unützer, RE Glasgow, MV Maciosek, and R Caucasianbird.
"Severity of Depression and Magnitude of Productivity Loss." *Annals of Family Medicine* 9, no.
4 (August 2011): 305–311.

Beck, Arne, A Lauren Crain, Leif I Solberg, Jürgen Unützer, Russell E Glasgow, Michael V
Maciosek, and Robin Caucasianbird. "Severity of Depression and Magnitude of Productivity
Loss." *Annals of Family Medicine* 9, no. 4 (August 2011): 305–311.

Bjelland, Ingvar, Steinar Krokstad, Arnstein Mykletun, Alv A. Dahl, Grethe S. Tell, and K. Tambs.
"Does a Higher Educational Level Protect Against Anxiety and Depression? The HUNT Study."
Social Science & Medicine 66, no. 6 (March 2008): 1334–1345.
doi:10.1016/j.socscimed.2007.12.019.

Boden, Joseph M., and David M. Fergusson. "Alcohol and Depression." *Addiction* 106, no. 5 (2011):
906–914. doi:10.1111/j.1360-0443.2010.03351.x.

"CDC - Workplace Health - Evaluation - Depression", n.d.
http://www.cdc.gov/workplacehealthpromotion/evaluation/topics/depression.html.

"CDC Data & Statistics | Feature: An Estimated 1 in 10 U.S. Adults Report Depression", n.d.
http://www.cdc.gov/Features/dsDepression/.

"CDC - Fact Sheets-Alcohol Use And Health - Alcohol." Accessed May 7, 2013.
http://www.cdc.gov/alcohol/fact-sheets/alcohol-use.htm.

Conner, Kyaien O, Valire Carr Copeland, Nancy K Grote, Daniel Rosen, Steve Albert, Michelle L
McMurray, Charles F Reynolds, Charlotte Brown, and Gary Koeske. "Barriers to Treatment and

Culturally Endorsed Coping Strategies Among Depressed African-American Older Adults."
Aging & Mental Health 14, no. 8 (November 2010): 971–983.

Conner, Kyaien O., Brenda Lee, Vanessa Mayers, Deborah Robinson, Charles F. Reynolds, Steve
Albert, and Charlotte Brown. "Attitudes and Beliefs About Mental Health Among African
American Older Adults Suffering from Depression." *Journal of Aging Studies* 24, no. 4
(December 1, 2010): 266–277.

Cook, Mary N, John Peterson, and Christopher Sheldon. "Adolescent Depression: An Update and
Guide to Clinical Decision Making." *Psychiatry (Edgmont (Pa.: Township))* 6, no. 9 (September
2009): 17–31.

"Current Depression Among Adults --- United States, 2006 and 2008", n.d.
http://www.cdc.gov/mmwr/preview/mmwrhtml/mm5938a2.htm?s_cid=mm5938a2_w.

De Wit, Leonore M, Annemieke van Straten, Marieke van Herten, Brenda W J H Penninx, and Pim
Cuijpers. "Depression and Body Mass Index, a U-shaped Association." *BMC Public Health* 9
(2009): 14. doi:10.1186/1471-2458-9-14.

Edlin, Mari. "Depression Can Be a Detriment to Workplace Productivity." ArticleStandard. *Managed
Healthcare Executive*, October 1, 2006.
http://managedhealthcareexecutive.modernmedicine.com/mhe/Disease+Management/Depression
-can-be-a-detriment-to-workplace-product/ArticleStandard/Article/detail/376838.

Ellermann, Caroline R, and Pamela G Reed. "Self-Transcendence and Depression in Middle-Age
Adults." *Western Journal of Nursing Research* 23, no. 7 (November 1, 2001): 698–713.

Essau, Cecilia A, Peter M Lewinsohn, John R Seeley, and Satoko Sasagawa. "Gender Differences in
the Developmental Course of Depression." *Journal of Affective Disorders* 127, no. 1–3
(December 2010): 185–190.

Fleming, Marc, Jamie C Barner, Carolyn M Brown, and Tawny Smith. "Treatment Disparities for Major Depressive Disorder: Implications for Pharmacists." *Journal of the American Pharmacists Association: JAPhA* 51, no. 5 (October 2011): 605–612.

Facilitated physical activity as a treatment for depressed adults: randomised controlled trial | BMJ. (n.d.). Retrieved February 12, 2013, from http://www.bmj.com/content/344/bmj.e2758?view=long&pmid=22674921

Gamble, James H P, Julian O M Ormerod, and Michael P Frenneaux. "Exercise Can Be Effective Therapy for Depression." *The Practitioner* 252, no. 1710 (September 2008): 19–20, 23–24.

Healthy People (2011, December). Healthy people 2020 summary of objectives. Retrieved from (http://www.healthypeople.gov/2020/topicsobjectives2020/pdfs/MentalHealth.pdf)

Healthy People (2011, December). Mental health and mental health disorders. Retrieved from (http://www.healthypeople.gov/2020/topicsobjectives2020/overview.aspx?topicid=28)

Illangasekare, Samantha, Jessica Burke, Geetanjali Chander, and Andrea Gielen. "The Syndemic Effects of Intimate Partner Violence, HIV/AIDS, and Substance Abuse on Depression Among Low-Income Urban Women." *Journal of Urban Health: Bulletin of the New York Academy of Medicine* (March 26, 2013). doi:10.1007/s11524-013-9797-8.

Kalibatseva, Zornitsa, and Frederick T. L. Leong. "Depression Among Asian Americans: Review and Recommendations." *Depression Research and Treatment* 2011 (2011): 1–9.

"ICD-10 Depression Diagnostic Criteria - General Practice Notebook." Accessed March 18, 2013. http://www.gpnotebook.co.uk/simplepage.cfm?ID=x20091123152205182440.

Lagerveld, SE, U Bültmann, RL Franche, F Van Dijk, MC Vlasveld, CM Feltz-Cornelis, DJ Bruinvels, et al. "Factors Associated with Work Participation and Work Functioning in

Depressed Workers: A Systematic Review." *Journal of Occupational Rehabilitation* 20, no. 3

(2010): 275–292.

Latino MH Facts_10 - Template.cfm." Accessed May 7, 2013.
http://www.nami.org/Template.cfm?Section=Fact_Sheets1&Template=/ContentManagement/Co
ntentDisplay.cfm&ContentID=99516.

Latzman, Robert D, James A Naifeh, David Watson, Jatin G Vaidya, Laurie J Heiden, John D

Damon, Terry L Hight, and John Young. "Racial Differences in Symptoms of Anxiety and

Depression Among Three Cohorts of Students in the Southern United States." *Psychiatry* 74, no.

4 (2011): 332–348.

Lee, Yunhwan, and Kyunghye Park. "Does Physical Activity Moderate the Association Between

Depressive Symptoms and Disability in Older Adults?" *International Journal of Geriatric

Psychiatry* 23, no. 3 (March 2008): 249–256.

Lewinsohn, P M, P Rohde, and J R Seeley. "Major Depressive Disorder in Older Adolescents:

Prevalence, Risk Factors, and Clinical Implications." *Clinical Psychology Review* 18, no. 7

(November 1998): 765–794.

Loneliness and Depression in Middle and Old Age: Are the Childless More Vulnerable? (n.d.).

Retrieved February 12, 2013, from

http://psychsocgerontology.oxfordjournals.org.ezproxy.gsu.edu/content/53B/6/S303

Lukachko, Alicia, and Mark Olfson. "Race and the Clinical Diagnosis of Depression in New Primary

Care Patients." *General Hospital Psychiatry* 34, no. 1 (February 2012): 98–100.

Marlowe, Joseph F. "Depression's Surprising Toll on Worker Productivity." *Employee Benefits

Journal* 27, no. 1 (March 2002): 16–21.

Marlowe, Joseph F. "Depression's Surprising Toll on Worker Productivity." *Employee Benefits

Journal* 27, no. 1 (March 2002): 16.

Michael Craig Miller. "Havard Mental Letter." *Havard Health Publications*, May 2011, 27 edition.

Mikkelsen, Stine Schou, Janne Schumann Tolstrup, Esben Meulengracht Flachs, Erik Lykke
    Mortensen, Peter Schnohr, and Trine Flensborg-Madsen. "A Cohort Study of Leisure Time
    Physical Activity and Depression." *Preventive Medicine* 51, no. 6 (December 2010): 471–475.

Nguyen, Ha T, and Alan B Zonderman. "Relationship Between Age and Aspects of Depression:
    Consistency and Reliability Across Two Longitudinal Studies." *Psychology and Aging* 21, no. 1
    (March 2006): 119–126.

"NHANES - About the National Health and Nutrition Examination Survey." Accessed March 20,
    2013. http://www.cdc.gov/nchs/nhanes/about_nhanes.htm.

"Older Adults: Depression and Suicide Facts (Fact Sheet)." *National Institute of Mental Health*, April
    2007. http://www.nimh.nih.gov/health/publications/older-adults-depression-and-suicide-facts-
    fact-sheet/index.shtml.

Ornelas, India J, and Krista M Perreira. "The Role of Migration in the Development of Depressive
    Symptoms Among Latino Immigrant Parents in the USA." *Social Science & Medicine (1982)* 73,
    no. 8 (October 2011): 1169–1177.

Physical activity and depress... [J Obstet Gynecol Neonatal Nurs. 2012] - PubMed - NCBI. (n.d.).
    Retrieved February 12, 2013, from http://www.ncbi.nlm.nih.gov/pubmed/22834847

"Physical Activity for Everyone: Guidelines: Adults | DNPAO | CDC", n.d.
    http://www.cdc.gov/physicalactivity/everyone/guidelines/adults.html.

"Physical Activity Statistics: Definitions | DNPAO | CDC." Accessed May 7, 2013.
    http://www.cdc.gov/nccdphp/dnpa/physical/stats/definitions.htm.

Physical activity status in adult... [Public Health Nurs. 2012 May-Jun] - PubMed - NCBI. (n.d.).
    Retrieved February 12, 2013, from http://www.ncbi.nlm.nih.gov/pubmed/22512422

Rethorst, Chad D, Bradley M Wipfli, and Daniel M Landers. "The Antidepressive Effects of Exercise: a Meta-analysis of Randomized Trials." *Sports Medicine (Auckland, N.Z.)* 39, no. 6 (2009): 491–511.

Schuch, F B, M P Vasconcelos-Moreno, C Borowsky, and M P Fleck. "Exercise and Severe Depression: Preliminary Results of an Add-on Study." *Journal of Affective Disorders* 133, no. 3 (October 2011): 615–618.

Skarupski, Kimberly A, Carlos F Mendes De Leon, Julia L Bienias, Lisa L Barnes, Susan A Everson-Rose, Robert S Wilson, and Denis A Evans. "African American–Caucasian Differences in Depressive Symptoms Among Older Adults Over Time." *The Journals of Gerontology Series B: Psychological Sciences and Social Sciences* 60, no. 3 (May 1, 2005): P136–P142.

Swendsen, J D, and K R Merikangas. "The Comorbidity of Depression and Substance Use Disorders." *Clinical Psychology Review* 20, no. 2 (March 2000): 173–189.

The Impact of Health Problems on Depression and Activities in Middle-Aged and Older Adults: Age and Social Interactions as Moderators. (n.d.). Retrieved February 12, 2013, from http://psychsocgerontology.oxfordjournals.org.ezproxy.gsu.edu/content/59/1/P19.short

Van de Velde, Sarah, Piet Bracke, and Katia Levecque. "Gender Differences in Depression in 23 European Countries. Cross-national Variation in the Gender Gap in Depression." *Social Science & Medicine (1982)* 71, no. 2 (July 2010): 305–313.

Van de Velde, Sarah, Piet Bracke, Katia Levecque, and Bart Meuleman. "Gender Differences in Depression in 25 European Countries After Eliminating Measurement Bias in the CES-D 8." *Social Science Research* 39, no. 3 (May 2010): 396–404.

Weisbord, Steven D, Linda F Fried, Mark L Unruh, Paul L Kimmel, Galen E Switzer, Michael J Fine, and Robert M Arnold. "Associations of Race with Depression and Symptoms in Patients on

Maintenance Haemodialysis." *Nephrology Dialysis Transplantation* 22, no. 1 (January 1, 2007): 203–208.

What Is Physical Activity? - NHLBI, NIH." Accessed April 27, 2013. http://www.nhlbi.nih.gov/health/health-topics/topics/phys/.

"WHO | Depression." *WHO*, n.d.

http://www.who.int/mental_health/management/depression/definition/en/.

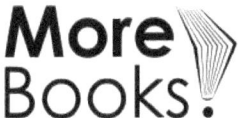
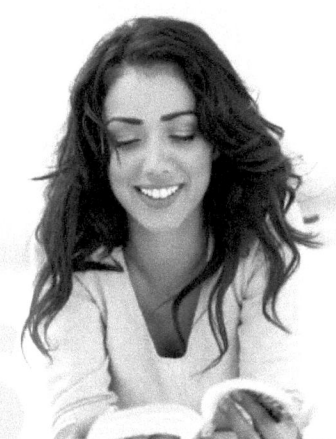

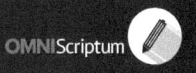

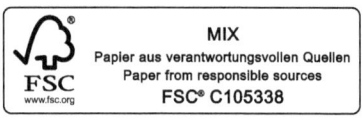

Printed by Books on Demand GmbH, Norderstedt / Germany